Smoothie For Weight Loss

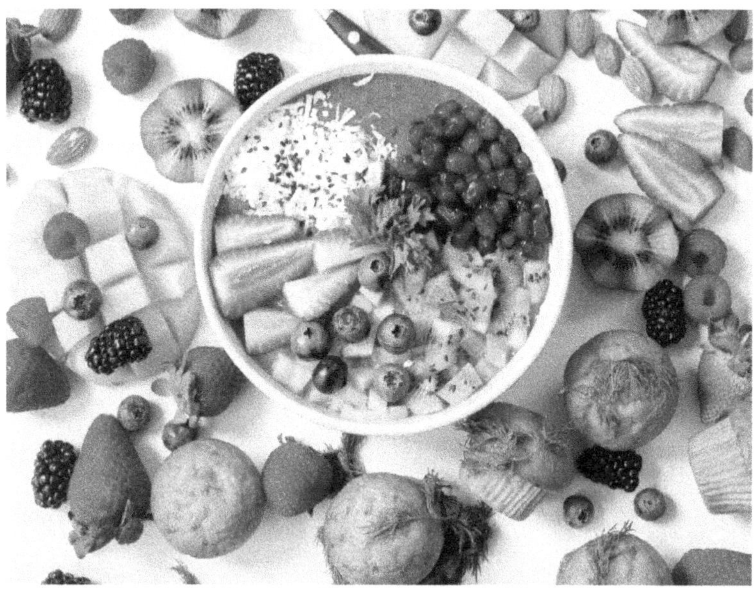

COMPLETE QUICK AND EASY 28 DAY SMOOTHIE PLAN FOR BEGINNERS

Emmanuel Scott

Copyright © by Emmanuel Scott 2023.

All rights reserved.

Before this document is duplicated or reproduced in any manner, the publisher's consent must be gained. Therefore, the contents within can neither be stored electronically, transferred, nor kept in a database. Neither in Part nor full can the document be copied, scanned, faxed, or retained without approval from the publisher or creator.

Table Of Contents

INTRODUCTION

COMPLETE 28-DAY SMOOTHIE PLAN

DAY 1:
BERRY BLAST
DAY 2:
GREEN GODDESS
DAY 3:
TROPICAL PARADISE
DAY 4:
PEACHY KEEN
DAY 5:
CITRUS SPLASH
DAY 6:
PROTEIN POWER
DAY 7:
CREAMY AVOCADO
DAY 8:
MIXED MELON
DAY 9:
BLUEBERRY BURST
DAY 10:
REFRESHING MINT
DAY 11:
STRAWBERRY DELIGHT
DAY 12:
CHERRY ALMOND
DAY 13:
CITRUS GREENS

DAY 14:
MANGO TANGO
DAY 15:
CHOCOLATE BANANA
DAY 16:
CREAMY BERRY
DAY 17:
PINEAPPLE COCONUT
DAY 18:
SPINACH APPLE
DAY 19:
KIWI LIME
DAY 20:
PEANUT BUTTER BANANA
DAY 21:
ORANGE CARROT
DAY 22:
RASPBERRY COCONUT
DAY 23:
MINTY WATERMELON
DAY 24:
VANILLA ALMOND
DAY 25:
BEET BERRY
DAY 26:
PINEAPPLE GINGER
DAY 27:
MIXED BERRY CHIA
DAY 28:
COCONUT MANGO

CONCLUSION

INTRODUCTION

In a small town plagued by unhealthy eating habits, Sarah, a determined individual seeking to conquer her weight struggles, discovered the incredible benefits of incorporating smoothies into her daily routine. With unwavering resolve, Sarah began substituting her unhealthy snacks with nutrient-rich smoothies, brimming with a medley of fruits, vegetables, and protein.

As time elapsed, Sarah witnessed a remarkable metamorphosis. The smoothies served as a catalyst for weight loss, appeasing her cravings while revving up her metabolism. The ample fiber content in the smoothies fostered prolonged satiety, effectively curbing mindless snacking. Moreover, the surge in energy levels and improved digestion fueled Sarah's capacity for intense workouts, resulting in the torching of excess calories.

Inspired by her personal triumph, Sarah emerged as a champion of healthy living within her community. She generously shared her prized smoothie recipes and fervently encouraged others to embark on the journey to wellness alongside her. The town rallied together, embracing the transformative power of smoothies as a key ally in weight loss and overall well-being. Through their collective efforts, the town blossomed into a vibrant, health-conscious community, with smoothies symbolizing vitality and self-care.

COMPLETE 28-DAY SMOOTHIE PLAN

Day 1:
Berry Blast

Ingredients:

1 cup mixed berries

1 banana

1 cup spinach

1 cup almond milk

1 tablespoon chia seeds

Preparation: Blend all the ingredients until smooth. Add ice cubes if desired.

Nutritional Value:

Calories: 230

Protein: 5g

Fat: 6g

Carbohydrates: 42g

Fiber: 12g

Day 2:
Green Goddess

Ingredients:

1 cup kale

1/2 cucumber

1/2 green apple

1 tablespoon lemon juice

1 cup coconut water

Preparation: Blend the ingredients until well combined. Depending on the needed consistency, add more water.

Nutritional Value:

Calories: 80

Protein: 3g

Fat: 1g

Carbohydrates: 19g

Fiber: 3g

Day 3:
Tropical Paradise
Ingredients:

1 cup pineapple

1/2 mango

1/2 banana

1 cup spinach

1 cup coconut milk

Preparation: Blend all the ingredients together until creamy and smooth.

Nutritional Value:

Calories: 210

Protein: 3g

Fat: 8g

Carbohydrates: 35g

Fiber: 6g

Day 4:
Peachy Keen

Ingredients:

1 cup peaches

1/2 cup Greek yogurt

1/2 cup almond milk

1 tablespoon honey

Preparation: Combine all the ingredients in a blender and blend until creamy.

Nutritional Value:

Calories: 240

Protein: 12g

Fat: 4g

Carbohydrates: 42g

Fiber: 3g

Day 5:
Citrus Splash

Ingredients:

1 orange

1/2 grapefruit

1/2 lemon

1 cup spinach

1 cup coconut water

Preparation: Squeeze the citrus fruits to extract the juice. Add the juice, spinach, and coconut water to a blender, and blend until well mixed.

Nutritional Value:

Calories: 120

Protein: 5g

Fat: 0g

Carbohydrates: 30g

Fiber: 5g

Day 6:
Protein Power

Ingredients:

1 scoop protein powder

1 banana

1 tablespoon almond butter

1 cup almond milk

Preparation: Blend each item together until it is smooth and creamy.

Nutritional Value:

Calories: 350

Protein: 30g

Fat: 13g

Carbohydrates: 34g

Fiber: 7g

Day 7:
Creamy Avocado

Ingredients:

1/2 avocado

1 cup spinach

1/2 banana

1 cup coconut milk

1 tablespoon flax seeds

Preparation: Blend all the ingredients until silky smooth.

Nutritional Value:

Calories: 290

Protein: 7g

Fat: 23g

Carbohydrates: 18g

Fiber: 10g

Day 8:
Mixed Melon

Ingredients:

1 cup mixed melon (watermelon, cantaloupe, honeydew)

1/2 cup Greek yogurt

1 tablespoon honey

1 cup coconut water

Preparation: The ingredients should be thoroughly blended.

Nutritional Value:

Calories: 150

Protein: 7g

Fat: 1g

Carbohydrates: 32g

Fiber: 1g

Day 9:
Blueberry Burst

Ingredients:

1 cup blueberries

1/2 banana

1 cup spinach

1 tablespoon almond butter

1 cup almond milk

Preparation: Blend all the ingredients until smooth and creamy.

Nutritional Value:

Calories: 250

Protein: 8g

Fat: 7g

Carbohydrates: 44g

Fiber: 10g

Day 10:
Refreshing Mint

Ingredients:

1 cup pineapple

1/4 cup fresh mint leaves

1/2 cucumber

1 tablespoon lime juice

1 cup coconut water

Preparation: Blend all the ingredients until well combined.

Nutritional Value:

Calories: 120

Protein: 3g

Fat: 0g

Carbohydrates: 30g

Fiber: 4g

Day 11:
Strawberry Delight

Ingredients:

1 cup strawberries

1/2 cup Greek yogurt

1/2 cup almond milk

1 tablespoon honey

Preparation: Blend all the ingredients together until smooth and creamy.

Nutritional Value:

Calories: 180

Protein: 10g

Fat: 3g

Carbohydrates: 30g

Fiber: 4g

Day 12:
Cherry Almond

Ingredients:

1 cup cherries

1 tablespoon almond butter

1/2 cup almond milk

1 tablespoon chia seeds

Preparation: Blend all the ingredients together until well combined.

Nutritional Value:

Calories: 230

Protein: 6g

Fat: 10g

Carbohydrates: 32g

Fiber: 6g

Day 13:
Citrus Greens

Ingredients:

1 orange

1/2 grapefruit

1 cup spinach

1/2 cucumber

1 cup coconut water

Preparation: Squeeze the citrus fruits to extract the juice. Add the juice, spinach, cucumber, and coconut water to a blender, and blend until well mixed.

Nutritional Value:

Calories: 110

Protein: 5g

Fat: 0g

Carbohydrates: 28g

Fiber: 5g

Day 14:
Mango Tango

Ingredients:

1 cup mango

1/2 banana

1 cup spinach

1 cup coconut milk

Preparation: Blend all the ingredients together until creamy and smooth.

Nutritional Value:

Calories: 210

Protein: 4g

Fat: 8g

Carbohydrates: 35g

Fiber: 6g

Day 15:
Chocolate Banana

Ingredients:

1 banana

1 tablespoon cocoa powder

1/2 cup Greek yogurt

1 cup almond milk

Preparation: Blend all the ingredients together until smooth and creamy.

Nutritional Value:

Calories: 280

Protein: 14g

Fat: 6g

Carbohydrates: 45g

Fiber: 8g

Day 16:
Creamy Berry

Ingredients:

1 cup mixed berries

1/2 cup Greek yogurt

1 tablespoon honey

1 cup coconut water

Preparation: Blend all the ingredients until well combined.

Nutritional Value:

Calories: 170

Protein: 10g

Fat: 0g

Carbohydrates: 35g

Fiber: 5g

Day 17:
Pineapple Coconut

Ingredients:

1 cup pineapple

1/2 cup coconut milk

1 tablespoon lime juice

1 tablespoon shredded coconut

Preparation: Blend all the ingredients together until smooth and creamy. Sprinkle shredded coconut on top before serving.

Nutritional Value:

Calories: 230

Protein: 2g

Fat: 13g

Carbohydrates: 29g

Fiber: 4g

Day 18:
Spinach Apple

Ingredients:

1 apple

1 cup spinach

1/2 banana

1 cup almond milk

1 tablespoon chia seeds

Preparation: Blend all the ingredients until smooth. Add ice cubes if desired.

Nutritional Value:

Calories: 200

Protein: 6g

Fat: 5g

Carbohydrates: 38g

Fiber: 10g

Day 19:
Kiwi Lime

Ingredients:

2 kiwis

1 tablespoon lime juice

1 cup spinach

1 cup coconut water

Preparation: Blend all the ingredients until smooth. Add ice cubes if desired.

Nutritional Value:

Calories: 140

Protein: 4g

Fat: 1g

Carbohydrates: 32g

Fiber: 8g

Day 20:
Peanut Butter Banana

Ingredients:

1 banana

1 tablespoon peanut butter

1/2 cup Greek yogurt

1 cup almond milk

Preparation: Blend all the ingredients together until smooth and creamy.

Nutritional Value:

Calories: 320

Protein: 15g

Fat: 11g

Carbohydrates: 44g

Fiber: 6g

Day 21:
Orange Carrot

Ingredients:

1 orange

1 carrot

1 cup spinach

1 cup coconut water

Preparation: Blend all the ingredients until well combined.

Nutritional Value:

Calories: 140

Protein: 5g

Fat: 1g

Carbohydrates: 32g

Fiber: 7g

Day 22:
Raspberry Coconut

Ingredients:

1 cup raspberries

1/2 cup coconut milk

1/2 banana

1 tablespoon honey

1 cup spinach

Preparation: Blend all the ingredients until smooth and creamy.

Nutritional Value:

Calories: 190

Protein: 4g

Fat: 6g

Carbohydrates: 35g

Fiber: 10g

Day 23:
Minty Watermelon

Ingredients:

2 cups watermelon

1/4 cup fresh mint leaves

1/2 cucumber

1 tablespoon lime juice

1 cup coconut water

Preparation: Blend all the ingredients until well combined.

Nutritional Value:

Calories: 100

Protein: 2g

Fat: 0g

Carbohydrates: 25g

Fiber: 3g

Day 24:
Vanilla Almond

Ingredients:

1 cup almond milk

1/2 teaspoon vanilla extract

1/4 cup rolled oats

1 tablespoon almond butter

1 tablespoon honey

Preparation: Blend all the ingredients together until smooth and creamy.

Nutritional Value:

Calories: 240

Protein: 6g

Fat: 10g

Carbohydrates: 34g

Fiber: 6g

Day 25:
Beet Berry

Ingredients:

1 small beetroot

1 cup mixed berries

1/2 banana

1 cup spinach

1 cup almond milk

Preparation: Blend all the ingredients until well combined.

Nutritional Value:

Calories: 180

Protein: 5g

Fat: 3g

Carbohydrates: 35g

Fiber: 8g

Day 26:
Pineapple Ginger

Ingredients:

1 cup pineapple

1-inch piece of ginger

1/2 banana

1 cup spinach

1 cup coconut water

Preparation: Blend all the ingredients until well combined.

Nutritional Value:

Calories: 170

Protein: 4g

Fat: 1g

Carbohydrates: 40g

Fiber: 5g

Day 27:
Mixed Berry Chia

Ingredients:

1 cup mixed berries

1 tablespoon chia seeds

1/2 cup Greek yogurt

1 cup almond milk

1 tablespoon honey

Preparation: Blend all the ingredients until smooth and creamy.

Nutritional Value:

Calories: 240

Protein: 11g

Fat: 6g

Carbohydrates: 36g

Fiber: 9g

Day 28:
Coconut Mango

Ingredients:

1 cup mango

1/2 cup coconut milk

1 tablespoon lime juice

1 tablespoon shredded coconut

Preparation: Blend all the ingredients together until smooth and creamy. Sprinkle shredded coconut on top before serving.

Nutritional Value:

Calories: 220

Protein: 3g

Fat: 13g

Carbohydrates: 32g

Fiber: 5g

CONCLUSION

In conclusion, "The 28-Day Smoothie Plan" offers a powerful and transformative journey towards better health and vitality. Through the incorporation of nutrient-rich ingredients and delicious smoothie recipes, this book provides a practical and sustainable approach to achieving weight loss goals.

By following the 28-day plan, readers will not only experience the benefits of shedding excess pounds but also witness improvements in energy levels, digestion, and overall well-being. The carefully crafted recipes offer a wide variety of flavors and combinations, ensuring that every day brings a new and exciting experience.

Moreover, the inclusion of preparation instructions and nutritional values empowers beginners to make informed choices and develop a deeper understanding of the impact of each ingredient on their health.

"The 28-Day Smoothie Plan" is not just a book; it's a roadmap to a healthier lifestyle. It encourages readers to embrace the power of wholesome, nourishing foods and embark on a transformative journey towards optimal well-being. So, grab your blender and get ready to sip your way to a happier, healthier you!.

www.ingramcontent.com/pod-product-compliance
Lightning Source LLC
Chambersburg PA
CBHW072343270726
48659CB00023B/2352